MW01269118

SCARY CRYPTID HORROR STORIES VOL 2

TABLE OF CONTENTS:

STORY 1

STORY 2

STORY 3

STORY 4

STORY 5

STORY 6

STORY 7

STORY 8

STORY 9

STORY 1

Kodiak is a tiny island off Alaska's coast where I spent much of my childhood. There is a town on the island, as well as a few settlements. You'll need to take a plane or boat to get there.

When I wasn't in class or working, I enjoyed hanging out with my friends, smoking weed, and hiking the nearby trails.

I decided it would be fun, on a regular day, to tease my buddy, who was already worried (A).

Stories of the "Agula'aq," pronounced "a-hole-uck," a creature very akin to a skinwalker, have been related by Native Alutiiq elders for generations.

Former humans who were shunned from their communities and were forced to resort to dark magic. Because these are considered taboo subjects, it's very rare to hear someone else's story about a similar situation.

I thought it would be hilarious to frighten the living daylights out of my buddy (A), so that's where the narrative begins. While we were wandering around the paths, I filled him in on all I knew about the being. At this point, nightfall has set in, and the four of us are feeling a little uneasy, so we decide to return to the vehicle.

As friend(A) drives us back, friend(B) requests if I can stop at the convenience store to pick up a pack of cigarettes for him; he's already got ten dollars in his room.

While waiting for him, my buddy (A) and I put on some tracks. To everyone's surprise, he quickly replies with, "I've just got 3 bucks. Maybe tomorrow, dude." It's OK, we shake hands and walk in the direction of my home so I can be dropped off.

While I'm relaxing on my bed, my friend(B) sends me a text message: "Where have you all disappeared to, anyway? I mistook the package for smokes. "

Hmm... With my response, I'm testing his memory to see whether he's forgotten our talk from ten minutes ago.

He insists that we weren't already gone when he went inside, ripped his room up looking for his money, and then ran outside to find us.

He thought we had abandoned him. I tell him I may be able to acquire his cigarettes for him nonetheless and go to his place to check if he's just messing with me. He continues to defend his account, and I have no reason to doubt it.

That guy wouldn't put his cigarettes before a practical joke. I'm trying to recall the topic of our conversation from the previous afternoon. We never mentioned it until now.

STORY 2

My grandma told us a story about a time in the late '50s when she was in the car with my grandmother and one of my uncles, Ron, who was only a toddler at the time, and they were driving southeast on a paved two-lane road lined with tiny trees and brush.

My grandmother said, as they rounded a turn while climbing a sequence of hairpins up a hill, "I reeked it before we discovered it." It stood there as they passed; it resembled a large hairy man except for the hairless areas on its lips and eyelids;

and, most intriguingly, its head sat atop its neck in an unusual manner as it turned its entire body to stare at them; its hair was brown and matted like a stray dog's.

When they had gone by, she looked back and saw it "step up out of the dump on the side of the road, and in one massive step it stepped all the way to the midpoint of the road, and in one further step it cleared the street into the ditch on the other side of the road, and within 3 stages it had cleared 10 meters into the mascara wand and trees and faded away from sight."

She said that her sister was clinging to her arm the whole time, sobbing and babbling like a raving lunatic, and that they would have both been sick in their chairs.

Ron, who was sitting in the back, slept through the whole thing.

STORY 3

In southeast Missouri, I visited a buddy at his lake home. In order to deal with the beavers or whatever was obstructing the drainage region, we drove a motorcycle with a travel trailer up and around the lake. Each of the four of us made up a full complement.

Two friends went on the ATV, while my other friend and I took the trailer. Leaving the ATV parked, we made our way to the water's edge on foot. From where we were walking, the two on the ATV lowered the weapon a short distance.

When my companion and I were standing approximately seventy-five yards away, we noticed something emerge from the woods and go toward the ATV. Its pure whiteness evoked an albino creature. The size was comparable to that of the ATV.

General appearance-wise, it resembled a lion, but its fluffy tail made it seem more like a werewolf or coyote. For 10 seconds, it sniffed around the ATV, gazed at us, and then sulked off into the woods.

I'm a big fan of the great outdoors, have spent considerable time inside the woods, and even achieved the rank of Eagle Scout, but

I've never experienced anything quite like it before or since. Someone would have probably heard about a white, mangy mountain lion if it had been living in a moderately crowded region

(there was a corner shop that was 5-10 minutes' drive from the lakehouse).

STORY 4

I've recounted this tale a million times, but it still gives me the creeps every time I recall what occurred to me when I was approximately 13 years old.

During the summer, my four best friends and I would spend every weekend camping in the woods belonging to one of our mutual acquaintances.

We found that Walmart had a two-pack of flares, and we used them to set things on fire whenever we felt like messing about and having some fun.

My buddy asked if he was using the flare to melt the handle and strike the machete with a hammer to distort it, and I said he could do anything he wanted with it since it was such a cheap machete that I didn't mind.

When he does, I hear somebody close by, and when I look, I see something that had to be at least 7-8 feet tall, but since it was night, all I saw was an eye moving through the shadows. Something seemed crimson as well, but that may have just been my strained eyes looking at the flare.

I stood up and said, "Guys," and no one understood me until a bush shook behind my pal.

We've huddled together out of sheer terror. My pal makes the executive decision to contact his mom and bail My buddy and I waited in the tent while the other three went to pick up our friend and return her to the road. Our group was resting in the tent when we heard noises outside and decided, "Okay, they're just messing with us."

To this day, I will never forget the day I was praying in a tent when I saw what looked like a fucking finger wandering up the side of the tent, nearly poking through it, on its way to the front.

When I asked my buddy, "Hey man, where you at?" I was expecting to hear him say something about being outside the tent. Instead, he replied that he was at home, which was just five minutes away from the camp site.

We never had something like that happen again, but it was the scariest thing I've ever experienced. I don't remember much else about that night, but I remember the entire situation very well.

STORY 5

So you know where I'm coming from. I was born and raised in Kentucky. great hunting opportunities, and I'm not the only one who appreciates the area's abundance of trees.

I didn't think the woods could possibly be home to any kind of mystery. I entertained the possibility that bigfoot existed, but I had my doubts. What transpired has convinced me that there is a mystery beyond our understanding.

Seeing as how Gander Mountain was closing down, I figured, "Why the fuck not?" and purchased a 60-round drum magazine for my newly acquired AR-15-style rifle (a Ruger AR556, if anybody cares).

After doing some research on the drums, I learned that they were fantastic and almost never had any problems (this will be important later). I chose to take it for a spin and adjust the sights on my rifle just several days after I received it. The downward spiral begins right here.

I've already mentioned that Kentucky is heavily forested. About three-quarters of the acreage I owned was covered in dense forest. In the woods, our cows had beaten out a few smaller routes in addition to the main one we used to drive our gator along.

I took a stroll down by the stream on a route partially cleaned by the cows. Our cattle live in a large field at the terminus of the trail, which I use to sight in my firearms when they are not around.

As soon as I stepped over the fence leading to the field, I had the uneasy feeling that I was being watched. I ignored it since I've gone back to that area several times and never had any problems.

So I just keep going, ignoring the sense that I'm being followed, but at the same time being aware of that sensation. I'm aware of the fact that I sense surveillance, but I wasn't paying any attention to it until today. It takes no more than two minutes to make your way to the area beside the stream.

As I proceeded deeper, the sensation that something was following me became stronger. The intensity of the sensation became intolerable about the time I was halfway there, and I had to give in to it. It occurred to me that the barrel magazine I was carrying was empty, so I paused to begin filling it. Since my main intention was to scope my rifle, I figured 20 rounds would be plenty.

Therefore, I have halted, am maintaining constant vigilance, and am now filling my magazine. When I first began loading rounds into the drum, I was hit by the odor of something that had been dead for a long time and had been left out in the sun to decay.

When I turned to look around, I saw the possum's skeletal remains directly behind me. That thing was ripped to shreds. That thing was almost waiting for me to locate it. It seemed to have been dead for little more than a day, but the odor suggested it had been dead for much longer. Because of my negative reaction, I loaded each magazine twice as fast.

There was still time to turn back when I saw the dead possum, but I blew it.

So, I made the choice to proceed. The thought that anything could go wrong back there made me think my mind was playing tricks on me, but it had always been perfectly safe.I saw it happen while I was walking to the field.

.

At the head of the stream, I felt like I was always being watched. I nearly reached the creek's outlet and the forest's edge when I heard a splash.

With my nerves on edge, I aimed my pistol in the direction of the sound, but there was no ammunition in the chamber. I'll never forget seeing her walk away from me down the stream bank.

They were at least 6–8 feet tall, and perhaps more. extremely thin. Now picture a fully grown guy who weighs just 120 pounds. Now, make him eight feet tall while his breadth remains the same. Bipedal gait, extremely long limbs.

Its skin was stretched tautly across its whole body.

Apart from the splash it produced as it stepped into the stream, it walked silently. It walked in an odd way, rather like a crawl, but with big steps. It may have been the muddy stream bank, however.

A light brown, nearly the shade of a deer, was also present. All I can recall at the moment is what I just wrote; if I recall anything more, I'll add it in.

That's why I feel if I'm being watched is clear to me now. All is set to fire a shot: the magazine is full and the bolt is cocked. Keep in mind that I have stated the publication to be very trustworthy. In case this monstrosity chooses to strike, I push the bolt release on my pistol and chamber a cartridge (I did not intend on striking first).

The bullet refuses to move from its fixed position in the magazine. That magazine had never been used previously by me, so it wasn't worn out from many loadings. Why didn't this magazine function when the power of a closing rifle bolt might crush your finger?

This item is the only thing I can think of that may have caused that. I had to send the magazine back to Magpul since it stopped functioning properly. Of course, I didn't tell them that; instead, I said the magazine had malfunctioned multiple times. However, let us return to the matter at hand.

The first shot, which is the simplest, got jammed. The creature quickly and silently leaves the area. A little introduction was all I needed to learn the information I shared.

Let's make some guesses now. A year ago, in late May, this occurred. I have all of the emails I had with Magpul about the drum, so I'm using them as a reference; after this, I really needed a solid foundation on which to build.

As for what the creature was, a friend of mine who knows more about these things than I do and I think it might have been a fucking Wendigo.

Everything I mentioned sounds like a Wendigo, which is why we assume they exist.

According to what I'd read, they're very slender and tall, give out a constant deathly odor (which would explain the possum's stink), are lightning quick, come in a variety of colors (including light brown), and sometimes resort to viciously killing other animals in order to intimidate people (again, the possum).

Its conduct was the one aspect for which we were at a loss. Exactly and I'm still here.

Wendigos have a reputation for being very violent. Nothing happened, but it kept an eye on me. Instead of attacking me or trying to talk to me, it ran away as if scared or trying to lead me to where it wanted to go.

Despite this, I have never seen it again. There have been other times when I've gone to a certain field and walked the same route, but I've never felt like I was being watched quite as intently as I did that day. I still believe that there is anything beyond our planet.

I've tried to convince myself that someone is watching me from the outside, but nothing comes close to that day.

Any other readers who have questions they'd want me to address may post them in the comments.

I need to get this off my chest, and talking about it will help. Please let me know if you have any insight on what I may have seen or if you have a more educated estimate. What really is in my woods?

I know this is a pretty long explanation, but I thought it necessary to give every little detail. The finer points highlight how completely screwed I might have been. There was a perfect storm of circumstances aimed towards fucking me.

Sorry, I failed to mention that there has been a sizable Native American population in my region. Every year, I unearth a great deal of flint, but it is the arrowheads that prove their presence.

Another likely starting point is a Highway of Tears location that is less than 5 miles from my house; I'm sure many of them grew desperate and started out on it.

STORY 6

I once encountered what was likely a boar after venturing far into the forest. Maybe not remarkable to most people, but terrifying to someone raised in a place where predatory creatures aren't a constant threat. Now, the concept that it may be anything vague is really mind-blowing.

(This isn't some terrifying ghost tale; it's simply a boring tale about a pig.)

I just returned from a trip to the middle of nowhere in France. The home backed up to a large forest. There was a narrow trail that went straight into the woods from the backyard. Animals that emerge from the nighttime forest create the pathway.

We wanted to go do some woodland adventuring with our younger brother. I was looking forward to sharing my impressions of the gorgeous forest with them, since I had previously visited a small portion of it.

There is just one rather short natural tunnel leading in from the end of the trail, which is incredibly thick. The two of us tiptoe into the tunnel.

Take precautions to avoid being pricked by the thorns. There is a rustling sound coming from the woods while we do this.

The presence of an animal in the area where we planned to go became apparent at this point. Unlike the rustling sounds I've heard from birds and squirrels, this one seemed like it was coming from a much larger animal in the forest.

We've decided to investigate to determine what kind of animal this is. There are additional sounds of rustling and footsteps as we get closer. At some point, there was a brief snort. I knew at that point that we were quite near to a wild boar.

In all my years, I've never ever seen a wild boar, much less come anywhere near one. although I am aware of the necessity for some caution on your part.

The boar was apparently very close to us because of the noises it was making, but we couldn't see it because of the thick foliage.

For a while, I was torn between wanting to stay and watch the boar and leaving immediately since I didn't want to encounter a hostile pig.

In the end, I was unable to see the boar. Even though I was perfectly quiet and moving extremely slowly, I spent at least ten minutes attempting to get a peek at it.

Not only did I fail to see it, but I also could not locate it. This thing that looked like it was right next to us could not be located. I made a couple more trips there, hoping to get a glimpse of a wild animal. There were no other people in the woods at those other times.

That pig could not have even been a boar.

STORY 7

Although I was living in Nevada at the time, every year during the summer break, my parents would transport me to see my grandparents at their cabin in the New Jersey pine barrens.

I was 8 years old when I left in 1982, never to return. It was late at night, perhaps after 11, my grandparents were in bed, and I was reading Archie comics by flashlight (and I still remember the exact issue I was on).

Being completely unfamiliar with it, it frightened the living daylights out of me. That cry wasn't made by a mountain lion or a coyote; I've heard both!

When I turn out the lights, the cabin is so silent that a mouse might urinate on a piece of cotton.

Once again, I hear the scream, and this time it seems like it's coming from directly outside my window.

I'm about to lose it when I hear what sounds like stones being flung or rolled on the roof and some sniffing or snuffling coming from outside the window. I'm not going to waste time looking; I'm rousing Grandpa right now.

After he registers my panic, he quickly takes the flashlight and begins a thorough sweep of the cabin's outside. When he returns, he claims he was unable to detect any sounds or sights.

Naturally, I end up spending the night in their bed. We checked beneath my window in the morning, and sure enough, there were fist-sized hoof tracks leading from the woods to my house. When I first saw the tracks outside my bedroom window, I assumed they were made by a wild pig or something similar.

However, when I was exploring on the opposite side of the house, I observed that there was another set of prints heading AWAY from the house, practically in a straight line from my window. When I told my dad (who had spent much of his childhood in the pine barrens) about what we had seen, he said, "Oh, it had to be the Jersey Devil." I had no idea what he meant at the time, but I'd never forgotten the incident.

When I was older, I spent a lot of time in the catalog reading literature about the Jersey Devil, and it sounded a lot like that to me.

Or, it may have been a pig... I'd like to believe it was a pig instead of a horse/goat/bat hybrid that was the cursed kid of a devil worshipper or some crap...

I never came back to Jersey to see the parents when they owned that awful cottage.

STORY 8

I have a lot of experience in the wilderness; I'm good at hunting, camping, trekking, and just plain survival.

I've spent a lot of time around animals, so when my cousin and I were attacked by what we now believe to be a dogman cryptid, it caught my attention because it didn't look like a bear or a normal wolf.

Bears and normal wolves can't run on two legs like this creature did, but it felt perfectly at home doing so. If you want further information, I can provide it.

It was probably in April or May of 2007, and I was about 17 years old and reasonably confident in my outdoor abilities at the time. When I was a kid, my family owned a cabin in northwest Wisconsin. I spent most of my summers there, so I have a deep familiarity with the area's woods.

However, it was always prudent to stay inside the cabin, or at the very least, near the beach bonfire, at night due to the presence of bears, grizzlies, and cougars. Bonfires were especially unnerving since the treeline could be seen from the camp fire and the beach, giving the impression that someone was watching you. Before this encounter, however, the woods during the daytime never looked out of the ordinary or eerie.

This occurred between 1300 and 1400, roughly. My cousin and I were engaged in an airsoft battle; I was dressed in full forest camouflage, while he was not; I withdrew along the ATV track into the trees for a tactical advantage; and the battle lasted from 200 meters to three-quarters of the way up the route.

At this point, we had had enough, and we were going to stand at the edge of such a clearing on the trail, talking, with him maybe ten meters from me, when I opted to play with him.

He froze, then I came to the realization the woods were dead silent, and I started checking the treeline and another edge of the emptying from left to right, and that's when I saw it.

It was as large as a black bear, at least 15 lbs, but not normal; it was on two legs, crouched next to a tree, with its arm clutching the tree, gripping with a clawed paw, and it had reddish brown fur, which gave it away when it started panting and looking at my cousin.

When I said, "We have to go," my cousin took off running. I returned my gaze to Wolfy, who had locked on, and ran a few measures on two feet before turning and running when Wolfy appeared to be on all fours.

The wolf eventually accused us and made it sound like we were right on our asses as we barreled through brush, but it let us go once we broke from the tree line and decided to head for the cabin.

The sheer scale of the thing resonated with me the most; while standing, Wolfy seemed to be about 7 feet tall, and where its paws should have been, it looked like it was holding its massive, clawed hands.

Now I really don't know how to rationalize it; I've heard wolves would sometimes kind of walk upright, but they can't sprint on two legs, wolves don't grow that large, and black bears basically waddle on two legs.

A werewolf or dogman is the most ridiculously close comparison. Your attention is appreciated.

STORY 9

When I was approximately 14 and lived in Montana, I saw something that resembled Cryptod. Due to our location on the outside of town, I often took lengthy walks late at night.

Whenever I passed a certain point on my regular walking path, something seemed odd. For some reason, there were maybe three empty spaces, and the asphalt turned to gravel just at the edges of the lots, and for some reason, it really freaked me out.

Not only did I despise passing by those empty lots, but so did everyone else I spoke with. These properties faced an empty canal on the opposite side of the road, which was approximately 20 feet wide.

One night, I took a stroll with a flashlight in hand since we lacked enough street lighting. I was nearing the road's edge and the commencement of the lots when my flashlight began to flicker and then die. Since the parking lots were hilly and curvy, I heard a truck speeding around one of the corners. A white vehicle with very bright headlights stopped on the dirt road in front of me.

If I hadn't seen the vehicle before, I would have assumed I was being abducted. The guy inside was so drowsy that I could tell he wasn't staring at me.

Once I turned back, I saw three huge wolf-like animals skulking from beneath a tree. In preparation for their strange hopping/dragging gait, each one of them leaned down and extended one enormous clawed hand.

They all followed the same path, which led them straight to the canal, where they vanished.

When I turned around, the driver had slammed on the throttle, sending the vehicle careening over the dirt. After a brief period of darkness, my flashlight turned back on. Instead of walking by those parking lots on my way home, I turned around and sprinted in the other direction.

Before I built my home, I discovered a pathway leading back into the towering cliffs. To the rear was a cave used by locals in search of a quiet drink.

There was a rustle in the bushes as I drove by, as well as another animal crossing the road at that spot. When I finally made it home and flung open the door, I heard a low growl behind me. As soon as I heard the sound of approaching footsteps, I dashed inside and quit taking walks at night.

Made in United States
Troutdale, OR
11/25/2023

14925643R00020